Acute and long-term stress sufferers: Are you at risk? Essential ways in managing it

by

Micheal L. Williamson

Table of Contents

Introduction

There is hardly any group of people that stress does not affect. It plagues the young or old, rich or poor, employer or employee, teacher or student, doctor or patient, mason or apprentice, male or female, parents or children. Additionally, it is connected to all forms of activity, and the only way to prevent it is to never do anything. However, stress is a necessary part of existence. Feelings joy, a tennis match, or an intriguing melodrama stresses us out. When we wake up in the morning, we are at our least stressed out—and we are aware of this. Mental disorientation and poor motor coordination are likely to occur. Stress makes us live and wakes us up. Problems develop when certain stress, either mental or physical, is applied for an extended period. "Many of us associate stress with everyday stresses or more serious ones like losing a partner or rising debt.

Many people associate the term with strain or pressure. It may resemble human stress in various respects. We must adjust to this physical or mental influence on our bodies to avoid injury. Some instances: On a hot day, you are outside in the sun. You become more heated. That kind of stress exists. Alternately, you exhaust yourself while playing a sport or gardening. Your muscles become fatigued as a result of a brief chemical imbalance in them. That is also stress. However, you have control mechanisms to offset such stress and return to a balanced state. Perspiration is one way your body cools itself. Another is getting a good night's rest, which enables your muscles to recover. Stress subsides. But nowadays, it's usual to associate stress with mental strain or tension, which can also cause physical changes. When we are unaware of the changes taking place within us, we might not be able to support our body's attempts at adaptation. Few people can say they have never experienced intense stress. The severity of our specific issues—money, family, sex, and crime—determines how acute the stress is. What best defines our time, according to a recent newspaper article, is not a particular acting or dressing style. The phrase "the horrible feeling of stress" is used to describe it. Unborn children are also affected. When pregnant women are under stress, such as from marital conflict or the fear of losing their employment, the unborn child may suffer physical, mental, or emotional impairment. Stress has the unfavourable side effect of causing more problems. As a result, many people miss work, which exacerbates their financial issues. It encourages violence even within marriage. There will always be some tension in life, which is neither healthy nor unhealthy. Stressful activities include getting out of bed in the morning and watching an exciting baseball game. Extreme, ongoing stress is damaging stress (or discomfort). Since many of the pressures we face are caused by other people or circumstances in our own lives, it makes sense that they may seem insurmountable. But is there anything we can do to prevent harmful stress? If we could properly manage stress, we could have fewer problems overall, including those that are harmful to our health. Acute and long-term stress sufferers: Are you at risk Essential ways in managing it, is a brilliantly titled book that discusses stress in detail, its causes, symptoms, and how to manage it.

Chapter one

Definition of stress

Stress is any physical, physiological, or emotional factor that causes strain on the body or mind. Another way to think of stress is as the body's natural response to a trying circumstance. In most cases, stress starts in the brain. It causes your body's hormones to function properly. It may cause a rise in breathing rate, a fall in blood pressure, and the ability of the lungs to expand or contract. "Broadly defined, stress is what happens to the body when it is subjected to anything," writes the author of teenage Stress. "Nervous strain, disease, cold, heat, damage, and so on."

Types or forms of stress

Stress can be classified according to the degree of its occurrence, besides this, it also occurs in various forms and kinds.

a) Acute (short-term) stress

The stresses of daily life are to blame for this. It frequently involves uncomfortable circumstances that need to be rectified. The stress may typically be managed because it is incidental and transient. Of course, some people seem to thrive on chaos; they seem to jump from one catastrophe to another. Even this extreme amount of acute stress is manageable. However, until he understands the impact his turbulent lifestyle is having on him and those around him, the sufferer may resist change. Acute stress, also known as "the good stress," is transient. This is so that they can accomplish their goals, put in more effort, or develop a talent, particularly if they are working or participating in an athletic event. A healthy amount of stress also shows that you are hard working and that your conscience is still active. Below are symptoms of acute stress.

i) Dry mouth

ii) Sweating

iii) Rapid breathing

iv) Faster heart rate

v) Tense muscles

 vi) Nausea

vii) Headaches

viii) Tooth grinding

b) Chronic (long-term) stress

Here, the victim sees no way out of a trying circumstance, whether it is the hardships of poverty or the unhappiness of a hated job—or no job at all. Ongoing familial issues might also cause chronic stress. Stress might also result from providing care for a sick relative. Whatever the cause, chronic wear down its victim day in and day out, week in and week out, month in and month out. One book on the issue claims that "the worst thing about chronic stress is that individuals get used to it."

Acute stress is immediately noticeable because it is fresh, whereas chronic stress is disregarded. After all, it is seasoned, well-known, and even comforting. Constant stress can result in cancers, diabetes, and stomach ulcers. The negative stress is this. When a certain stress, either mental or physical, is applied for an extended period of time, difficulties result. This kind of stress has an impact on the victim's physical, emotional, and mental health. People may use medications or even binge drink to cope with this type of stress. It affects how we interact with other people. It is defined by the following effects:

i) affects the Nervous system causing: irritability, anxiety, depression, insomnia/tiredness, and headache.

ii) inappropriate eating habits

iii) sexual disorders: impotence disrupted menstrual cycle

iv) aches and pains

v) increased sickness frequency

vi) it can cause cholesterol to accumulate in the arteries or produce hardening of the arteries. An example is High blood pressure, Stroke,

vii) affects the endocrine system causing diabetes, lowered immunity, increased illness, mood swings, and weight gain. White blood cells and the lymphatic system may be hampered, impairing the body's capacity to fight disease and respond to foreign substances.

viii) ulcers.

Here, the victim sees no way out of a trying circumstance, whether it is the hardships of poverty or the unhappiness of a hated job—or no job at all. Ongoing familial issues might also cause chronic stress. Stress might also result from providing care for a sick relative.

c) Traumatic stress

This kind of stress develops as a result of the effects of a terrible catastrophe, like a rape, an accident, or a natural disaster. This kind of stress affects a lot of combat veterans and survivors of concentration camps. Vivid memories of the trauma, even years later, as well as enhanced sensitivity to trivial incidents, are possible symptoms of traumatic stress. The patient may occasionally be identified as having post-traumatic stress disorder (PTSD).

Some claim that the amount and type of stress we have experienced in the past has a significant impact on how we react to stress in the present. According to some theories, traumatic experiences can change the chemical "wiring" of the brain, making a person far more susceptible to stress in the future. Of course, a person's response to stress can also be influenced by a variety of other factors, such as his physical make-up and the tools he has at his disposal to deal with difficult situation.

Chapter two
Causes of stress

The following things can make someone stressed out. They consist of:

a) Routine demands;

b) Financial or other insecurity.

c) Interpersonal disputes

d) A distressing event

Usefulness of stress

 Sometimes, a little tension and strain may be beneficial. A small bit of stress while working on a job or assignment inspires us to work hard and efficiently. Only when stress is extreme or poorly managed do its negative effects become apparent.

The truth is that you require stress—at least to some extent. Stress is helpful in emergencies.

ii) You require tension to carry out daily chores.

Everybody is constantly under stress to some extent. Dr. Hans Selye asserts that the best way to escape stress is to pass away.

Symptoms of stress

Some common indications of extreme stress or tension include the following:

i) Unusual irritability: Others have seen and even noted that you appear to become angry or irritated more frequently.

ii) Sleep problems: You struggle to get asleep, have trouble staying asleep, or wake up more frequently than normal.

iii) Changed breathing: You notice yourself developing a pattern of short, shallow breathing for no apparent cause.

iv) Muscle stiffness: Not related to exercise or productive activity.

v) Abdominal ache or discomfort: May be accompanied by a loss of appetite or the inability to eat more than a few small nibbles at once.

vi) Excitation: Changes in usual behaviours, such as becoming a nonstop talker who easily trembles or shivers at the slightest event.

It is important to remember that experiencing even one of these symptoms is a sign of extreme stress, which is bad for our health. Insufficient exercise, strained muscles from improper lifting, or both can result in back problems. If someone eats immediately before bed or drinks coffee or tea in the evening, they might have trouble sleeping. However, if you experience numerous of these signs and symptoms without a clear cause, you might be concerned that you are experiencing negative stress.

Effect of stress on the human body

i) Health disorders

ii) Emotional exhaustion

iii) Sleep problems

iv) Depression

v) Deteriorating relationship

Ailments caused by stress

i) Allergies

ii) Arthritis

iii) Asthma

iv) back, neck, and shoulder pain

v) colds

vi) depression

vii) diarrhea

viii) flu

ix) gastrointestinal problems

x) headaches

xi) heart problems

xii) insomnia

xiii) migraine

xiv) peptic ulcers

xv) sexual dysfunction

xvi) skin problems

Conditions in life that can cause stress

i) Spouse passing away

ii) Divorce

iii) Separation

iv) Jail time

v) Death of a close relative

vi) Injuries or illnesses

vii) Marital

viii)Workplace firing

ix) Marriage reconciliation

x) Retirement

xi) A family member's health has altered

xii) Pregnancy

xiii) Sexual difficulties

xiv) Adding a new family member

xv) Gaining a new family member.

xvi) Business reorientation.

Different parts of the human body that stress affects and its effects

Part of the body	Effect when stressed
Lungs	There is faster and increased breathing
Liver	Liver increases the blood's sugar content. Introduces sugar and fats into blood
Stomach	Digestion slows down
Eyes	The pupils always dilate
Muscles	It becomes tense, ready for action
Adrenal glands	powerful hormone like **cortisone and adrenaline** released into the blood stream
Heart	Prompts heartbeat, tightens blood vessels, and raises blood pressure

Chapter three

Management of stress

Lifting weights is a good way to deal with stress. A weight lifter needs to do proper pre-workout preparation to succeed. He accurately picks up the weights and doesn't load the bar with more weight than he can bear. Such actions allow him to develop strong muscles without endangering his body. However, if he doesn't follow these instructions, he risked tearing a muscle or perhaps breaking a bone. Similar to this, you can successfully handle the stresses you experience and complete the work you need to do without endangering yourself.

Some people use alcohol, drugs, or tobacco as a coping mechanism for persistent stress. Others start engaging in abnormal eating habits or passively sit in front of a computer or TV—habits that do not address the root cause but may even make it worse. According to the National Institutes of Health (NIH) in the United States, changing one's lifestyle is the greatest place to start when trying to reduce stress. "Begin by maintaining a balanced, healthy diet and making sure you're receiving enough rest and exercise. Limit your intake of caffeine and alcohol and abstain from cocaine, nicotine, and other illicit substances. The NIH also advises taking breaks from work, spending time with family and friends, developing your creative skills, and picking up an instrument. Here are some practical steps to follow:

1) Set clear and reasonable standards for yourself/ Reduce irritants

Don't expect to be perfect; instead, set reasonable expectations for both you and the people you come into contact with. But avoid being a stickler for accuracy. For anyone to carry, perfectionism is a stressful burden.

2. Live each day at a time/Adjust Your Viewpoint

Because every day brings its own set of worries, this is essential. The uneasiness of the present day would intensify if one worried about tomorrow. Where you live, how you live, or how you work is not the most crucial factors in how you deal with stress. It's also unrelated to how much you work out or sleep. It depends on how you perceive issues or stresses in life. You must develop the ability to assess your life's priorities. You may be in a stressful scenario due to a new job, a social event, the birth of a kid, or needing to take out a loan to make a significant purchase. A good question to ask yourself before acting or responding is, "Am I willing to accept the stress involved?" Does it merit it? How critical is this to my life? You'll become a happier person as a result of this rational appraisal, which will help you recognize your limitations and priorities.

3. Identify the specific cause of the stress

Keep in mind that stress arises when a psychological or physical issue keeps the body and mind on constant, but not necessarily high-level, alert. In many instances, all that is required to resolve the psychological and physical issues is their identification; then, without a doubt, the tension will go away. The point is that even if the cause of your stress cannot be prevented, your reaction to it will probably be less severe if you can identify it clearly in your mind. Knowing the source of the stress will help you manage it better. Find several strategies to handle the tension and get rid of it entirely.

4. Carry out a survey (research)

For instance, if you are stressed out by a large amount of schoolwork or a particular task, do some study on how to carry it out properly and with little to no stress. Ask those with experience who have already been through this time and challenge for their assistance.

5. Be fully organized/Set limits on some activities

Be organized to succeed. People who have good time management skills are significantly better able to handle stress. Prioritize the tasks that need to be done first to arrange. Next, create a schedule to ensure that things are not overlooked. Attempt to avoid putting things off. If you ignore problems, very few of them will go away. Instead, they typically get worse, adding to your tension. Do not wait to act once you have determined how you will handle a specific stressor. Do it immediately. Be practical and set up an acceptable schedule. Make a list of your daily tasks and complete them one at a time. Together with your parents, come up with a schedule for when and how to handle household chores. Do these then voluntarily and joyfully. Avoid engaging in risky, stressful activities that put you in uncomfortable or terrifying situations. It may be thrilling in the short term, but damaging in the long run.

6) Live a balanced life of work and play

This is something you can accomplish by choosing a job that you can realistically do. To reduce stress, pick a job that allows you to take breaks frequently. Use social media instead of spending a lot of time watching television. A person who consistently pushes themselves to their limits emotionally and physically is a prime risk for depression and burnout. Balance is the secret. Be trained to say no to requests that are too much for you to manage. Stretching is a great way to periodically "play" while you are working. By relaxing your face, neck, shoulders, and back muscles, you can reduce any tension building. However, schedule downtime in the same manner as work. Schedule some leisure time, perhaps with a pastime that will occupy you and keep your attention off the mental or emotional sources of your stress. In most cases, switching from one activity to another is more calming than complete rest, says Dr. Selye.

7. Try to Adapt

Some people make an effort to avoid the majority of stressful situations. For instance, people might relocate their homes or places of employment to avoid stressful situations, such as working in a stuffy or noisy environment or living in a congested, filthy metropolis.

That might be beneficial, but reducing stress does not necessarily require such extreme steps. For instance, some commuters depart earlier or later to lessen the stress of travelling on congested buses or roadways. They productively read, research, or compose letters while they are waiting. However, more crucially, individuals develop a sense of control over their life as a result of adapting in this way, which experts say is essential for managing stress.

8. Maintain good health by taking good care of yourself

You can accomplish this by paying attention to your diet. Proteins, produce, grains, fruits, and dairy products are all components of a balanced diet. Saturated fats and processed white wheat should be avoided. Intake of salt, refined sugar, alcohol, and caffeine should all be monitored. If you change your diet, you might become less sensitive to stress. Skip the fast food and excessive drinking.

Engage in regular exercise. Physical training is advantageous. Regular, moderate exercise—some advise three times a week—improves circulation, lowers cholesterol, and lowers your risk of having a heart attack. More importantly, exercise enhances feelings of well-being, possibly as a result of the endorphins released after hard exertion.

Get enough sleep. Lack of sleep makes you tired and makes it harder to control your tension. Try adhering to a normal bedtime and wake-up schedule if you have problems falling asleep. Some people advise limiting naps to 30 minutes to avoid disrupting a restful night's sleep. Avoid developing a routine of staying up late to engage in conversation over a cup of coffee or to watch a TV show, possibly a comedy or "talk show," which they claim helps them unwind. Any purportedly soothing impact must be evaluated against the potential accumulation of ongoing sleep debt. Lack of sleep puts stress on the body and mind and makes it harder to handle further stress. You can understand why it is crucial to obtain enough rest and sleep since stress results in physical changes in the body. Your body can heal itself as you sleep, re-establishing a healthy biochemical state. Therefore, if you suffer from stress, try getting more sleep, particularly by developing a regular sleep schedule week in and week out.

9. Choose important activities

Always prioritize your to-do list, clock how much time it takes to complete each item, and arrange breaks in between tasks.

10. Meditation

Take mental exercises every so often to assist you to concentrate your thoughts and energy.

11. Be positive and reduce the fear of failure

Anyone can experience stress from school tests. However, if you plan, have things in order the day before, go to bed early, and get enough sleep, you can reduce your fear of failing. Avoid using stimulants. They might make you anxious rather than calm you down. Take it easy, but try your best. Please keep in mind that a person is rarely made or broken by one test.

There will be other chances if you don't succeed. Keep a positive outlook.

12. Maintain Healthy Relationships

Try to enlist help in all you do. Having a social network offers at least some protection against becoming overloaded during difficult situations. A difference can be made by finding just one reliable person to confide in.

Dispute resolution. It makes sense to resolve conflicts promptly rather than letting anger fester. Any intensely negative emotion that causes a rush in stress hormones in the body, such as anger, appears to be the most powerful factor. Create family time. The resulting relationship encouraged family unity, which is severely absent nowadays. One study found that some working couples only spend 3.5 minutes a day playing with their kids on average. But when you're under stress, your family may be a great asset. According to a stress management book, "Family provides you an unconditional charter membership in an emotional support group that genuinely knows you for who you are and likes you anyhow." "One of the finest ways to reduce stress is family teamwork."

13. Talk out Stress

Don't bottle up all of your worries and problems. You'll feel a lot better after "getting it off your chest." Talk about it with a sympathetic friend you respect who might be able to offer assistance or guidance. Naturally, you don't want to be—and you shouldn't be—a whiner or complainer about problems, real or not. However, you do not become such by speaking to a reliable buddy. Beyond only feeling better emotionally, you might also gain a fresh perspective on your issues by making use of the useful advice of a more experienced individual.

14: Talk to a professional for help and support

In times like this, people are more important than ever. You should talk to someone if you are feeling overly anxious or worried. Talk to a trusted friend or relative about the stressors; express your feelings to the expert. Use the advice provided, get assistance, and divide labour. It may be wise to seek medical advice from a healthcare expert if your stress is continuous or severe enough to harm your health. Even the most powerful weightlifter has limitations. You concur. You don't have to bear the burden alone, though. Request their advice,

then use it.

Conclusion

Stress alone has the potential to have a significant medical impact on the immune system. Therefore, it cannot be dogmatically assumed that anybody who experiences stress, especially in its chronic form, would get a disease. On the other hand, it is unwise to deny medical care because of the mistaken belief that sickness can be willed away via optimism and positive thinking. Neither can it be stated that the absence of stress will guarantee good health. Therefore, it is important to understand that a disease's root cause is rarely limited to a single element. However, the link between stress and disease highlights the need of knowing how to manage this "slow poison" whenever possible. So let's say it again: Stress cannot be removed. However, you can learn to mitigate it.